If Lost, Please Return This Half Marathon Training Tracker To:

_____

Phone:_____

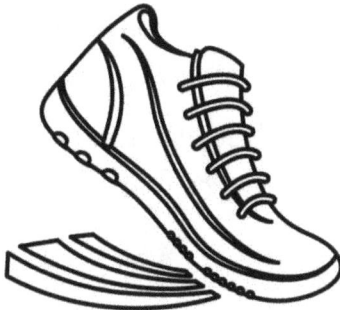

Tough Runs Don't Last
Tough Runners Do

DEDICATION

This Half Marathon Training Log book is dedicated to all the energetic and hard working people out there who love to run in marathons and want to document the process.

You are my inspiration for producing books and I'm honored to be a part of keeping all of your Half Marathon Training notes and records organized.

This journal notebook will help you record your details about your Half Marathon Training plan.

Thoughtfully put together with these sections to record: Race Details, Sample 12 Week Training Schedule, Personal Training Schedule, Daily Running Pages, Today's Goals, The Run, Notes & Thoughts and Reflection Notes

How to Use this Pizza Review Log Book:

The purpose of this book is to keep all of your Half Marathon notes all in one place. It will help keep you organized.

This Half Marathon Log Journal will allow you to accurately document every detail about your Half Marathon plan. It's a great way to chart your course through a memorable race.

Here are examples of the prompts for you to fill in and write about your experience in this book:

1. Race Details - Write Race Training for, Date of the Race, Date Registration Due, Entry Fee, Date to Start Training, Training & Race Goals.
2. Sample 12 Week Training Schedule - Gives you an example of what your training schedule could look like.
3. Personal Training Schedule - Write your own Personal Training Schedule to fit your own training needs.
4. Daily Running Pages - 12 Weeks (3 months) of Daily Running pages. Write date and day until the race.
5. Today's Goals - Record your Goals for the day including Distance, Speed & Other.
6. The Run - Prompts for writing Route, Weather Conditions, Start Time, End Time, Total Time, Total Distance and Average Pace.
7. Notes & Thoughts - Blank lined notes and personal thoughts for writing any other info you will want to write such as asthma condition, tracking soreness, favorite inspirational quote, results, etc.
8. Reflection Notes - Space to look back and reflect on what worked, anything you need to stop doing or do less of, what you think you need to do more of next time, what you worry about, did you get better or see improvements, etc.

Enjoy!

Race I'm Training For:

Date Of Race:

Date Registration Is Due:

Entry Fee:

Date I Need To Start Training:

TRAINING & RACE GOALS:

Sample 12-Week Training Schedule

	M	T	W	Th	F	S	S	Total
Week 1	2 miles	X Train	2 miles	Rest	1 mile	3 miles	Rest	
Week 2	2 miles	X Train	3 miles	Rest	1 mile	4 miles	Rest	
Week 3	2 miles	X Train	3 miles	Rest	2 miles	4 miles	Rest	
Week 4	2 miles	X Train	4 miles	Rest	2 miles	6 miles	Rest	
Week 5	3 miles	X Train	4 miles	Rest	2 miles	6 miles	Rest	
Week 6	3 miles	X Train	5 miles	Rest	2 miles	8 miles	Rest	
Week 7	3 miles	X Train	5 miles	Rest	3 miles	8 miles	Rest	
Week 8	3 miles	X Train	6 miles	Rest	3 miles	10 miles	Rest	
Week 9	4 miles	X Train	6 miles	Rest	3 miles	12 miles	Rest	
Week 10	4 miles	X Train	6 miles	Rest	2 miles	10 miles	Rest	
Week 11	3 miles	X Train	4 miles	Rest	2 miles	6 miles	Rest	
Week 12	2 miles	X Train	2 miles	Rest	Rest	Race Day	Rest	

My Training Schedule

	M	T	W	Th	F	S	S	Total
Week 1								
Week 2								
Week 3								
Week 4								
Week 5								
Week 6								
Week 7								
Week 8								
Week 9								
Week 10								
Week 11								
Week 12								

Date:_____ Days Till Race:_____

TODAY'S GOALS

Distance:

Speed:

Other:

THE RUN

Route:

Weather Conditions:

Time Start: Time End: Total Time:

Total Distance: Avg. Pace:

NOTES/THOUGHTS:

Date:_____ Days Till Race:_____

TODAY'S GOALS

Distance:

Speed:

Other:

THE RUN

Route:

Weather Conditions:

Time Start: Time End: Total Time:

Total Distance: Avg. Pace:

NOTES/THOUGHTS:

Date:_____ Days Till Race:_____

TODAY'S GOALS

Distance:

Speed:

Other:

THE RUN

Route:

Weather Conditions:

Time Start: Time End: Total Time:

Total Distance: Avg. Pace:

NOTES/THOUGHTS:

Date:_____ Days Till Race:_____

TODAY'S GOALS

Distance:

Speed:

Other:

THE RUN

Route:

Weather Conditions:

Time Start: Time End: Total Time:

Total Distance: Avg. Pace:

NOTES/THOUGHTS:

Date:_____ Days Till Race:_____

TODAY'S GOALS

Distance:

Speed:

Other:

THE RUN

Route:

Weather Conditions:

Time Start: Time End: Total Time:

Total Distance: Avg. Pace:

NOTES/THOUGHTS:

Date:_____ Days Till Race:_____

TODAY'S GOALS

Distance:

Speed:

Other:

THE RUN

Route:

Weather Conditions:

Time Start: Time End: Total Time:

Total Distance: Avg. Pace:

NOTES/THOUGHTS:

Date:_____ Days Till Race:_____

TODAY'S GOALS

Distance:

Speed:

Other:

THE RUN

Route:

Weather Conditions:

Time Start: Time End: Total Time:

Total Distance: Avg. Pace:

NOTES/THOUGHTS:

Date:_____ Days Till Race:_____

TODAY'S GOALS

Distance:

Speed:

Other:

THE RUN

Route:

Weather Conditions:

Time Start: Time End: Total Time:

Total Distance: Avg. Pace:

NOTES/THOUGHTS:

Date:_____ Days Till Race:_____

TODAY'S GOALS

Distance:

Speed:

Other:

THE RUN

Route:

Weather Conditions:

Time Start: Time End: Total Time:

Total Distance: Avg. Pace:

NOTES/THOUGHTS:

Date:_____ Days Till Race:_____

TODAY'S GOALS

Distance:

Speed:

Other:

THE RUN

Route:

Weather Conditions:

Time Start: Time End: Total Time:

Total Distance: Avg. Pace:

NOTES/THOUGHTS:

Date:_____ Days Till Race:_____

TODAY'S GOALS

Distance:

Speed:

Other:

THE RUN

Route:

Weather Conditions:

Time Start: Time End: Total Time:

Total Distance: Avg. Pace:

NOTES/THOUGHTS:

Date:_____ Days Till Race:_____

TODAY'S GOALS

Distance:

Speed:

Other:

THE RUN

Route:

Weather Conditions:

Time Start: Time End: Total Time:

Total Distance: Avg. Pace:

NOTES/THOUGHTS:

Date:_____ Days Till Race:_____

TODAY'S GOALS

Distance:

Speed:

Other:

THE RUN

Route:

Weather Conditions:

Time Start: Time End: Total Time:

Total Distance: Avg. Pace:

NOTES/THOUGHTS:

Date:_____ Days Till Race:_____

TODAY'S GOALS

Distance:

Speed:

Other:

THE RUN

Route:

Weather Conditions:

Time Start: Time End: Total Time:

Total Distance: Avg. Pace:

NOTES/THOUGHTS:

Date:_____ Days Till Race:_____

TODAY'S GOALS

Distance:

Speed:

Other:

THE RUN

Route:

Weather Conditions:

Time Start: Time End: Total Time:

Total Distance: Avg. Pace:

NOTES/THOUGHTS:

Date:_____ Days Till Race:_____

TODAY'S GOALS

Distance:

Speed:

Other:

THE RUN

Route:

Weather Conditions:

Time Start: Time End: Total Time:

Total Distance: Avg. Pace:

NOTES/THOUGHTS:

Date:_____ Days Till Race:_____

TODAY'S GOALS

Distance:

Speed:

Other:

THE RUN

Route:

Weather Conditions:

Time Start: Time End: Total Time:

Total Distance: Avg. Pace:

NOTES/THOUGHTS:

Date:_____ Days Till Race:_____

TODAY'S GOALS

Distance:

Speed:

Other:

THE RUN

Route:

Weather Conditions:

Time Start: Time End: Total Time:

Total Distance: Avg. Pace:

NOTES/THOUGHTS:

Date:_____ Days Till Race:_____

TODAY'S GOALS

Distance:

Speed:

Other:

THE RUN

Route:

Weather Conditions:

Time Start: Time End: Total Time:

Total Distance: Avg. Pace:

NOTES/THOUGHTS:

Date:_____ Days Till Race:_____

TODAY'S GOALS

Distance:

Speed:

Other:

THE RUN

Route:

Weather Conditions:

Time Start: Time End: Total Time:

Total Distance: Avg. Pace:

NOTES/THOUGHTS:

Date:_____ Days Till Race:_____

TODAY'S GOALS

Distance:

Speed:

Other:

THE RUN

Route:

Weather Conditions:

Time Start: Time End: Total Time:

Total Distance: Avg. Pace:

NOTES/THOUGHTS:

Date:_____ Days Till Race:_____

TODAY'S GOALS

Distance:

Speed:

Other:

THE RUN

Route:

Weather Conditions:

Time Start:　　　　　Time End:　　　　　Total Time:

Total Distance:　　　　　Avg. Pace:

NOTES/THOUGHTS:

Date:_____ Days Till Race:_____

TODAY'S GOALS

Distance:

Speed:

Other:

THE RUN

Route:

Weather Conditions:

Time Start: Time End: Total Time:

Total Distance: Avg. Pace:

NOTES/THOUGHTS:

Date:_____ Days Till Race:_____

TODAY'S GOALS

Distance:

Speed:

Other:

THE RUN

Route:

Weather Conditions:

Time Start: Time End: Total Time:

Total Distance: Avg. Pace:

NOTES/THOUGHTS:

Date:_____ Days Till Race:_____

TODAY'S GOALS

Distance:

Speed:

Other:

THE RUN

Route:

Weather Conditions:

Time Start: Time End: Total Time:

Total Distance: Avg. Pace:

NOTES/THOUGHTS:

Date:_____ Days Till Race:_____

TODAY'S GOALS

Distance:

Speed:

Other:

THE RUN

Route:

Weather Conditions:

Time Start: Time End: Total Time:

Total Distance: Avg. Pace:

NOTES/THOUGHTS:

Date:_____ Days Till Race:_____

TODAY'S GOALS

Distance:

Speed:

Other:

THE RUN

Route:

Weather Conditions:

Time Start: Time End: Total Time:

Total Distance: Avg. Pace:

NOTES/THOUGHTS:

Date:_____ Days Till Race:_____

TODAY'S GOALS

Distance:

Speed:

Other:

THE RUN

Route:

Weather Conditions:

Time Start: Time End: Total Time:

Total Distance: Avg. Pace:

NOTES/THOUGHTS:

Date:_____ Days Till Race:_____

TODAY'S GOALS

Distance:

Speed:

Other:

THE RUN

Route:

Weather Conditions:

Time Start: Time End: Total Time:

Total Distance: Avg. Pace:

NOTES/THOUGHTS:

Date:_____ Days Till Race:_____

TODAY'S GOALS

Distance:

Speed:

Other:

THE RUN

Route:

Weather Conditions:

Time Start: Time End: Total Time:

Total Distance: Avg. Pace:

NOTES/THOUGHTS:

Date:_____ Days Till Race:_____

TODAY'S GOALS

Distance:

Speed:

Other:

THE RUN

Route:

Weather Conditions:

Time Start: Time End: Total Time:

Total Distance: Avg. Pace:

NOTES/THOUGHTS:

Date:_____ Days Till Race:_____

TODAY'S GOALS

Distance:

Speed:

Other:

THE RUN

Route:

Weather Conditions:

Time Start: Time End: Total Time:

Total Distance: Avg. Pace:

NOTES/THOUGHTS:

Date:_____ Days Till Race:_____

TODAY'S GOALS

Distance:

Speed:

Other:

THE RUN

Route:

Weather Conditions:

Time Start: Time End: Total Time:

Total Distance: Avg. Pace:

NOTES/THOUGHTS:

Date:_____ Days Till Race:_____

TODAY'S GOALS

Distance:

Speed:

Other:

THE RUN

Route:

Weather Conditions:

Time Start: Time End: Total Time:

Total Distance: Avg. Pace:

NOTES/THOUGHTS:

Date:_____ Days Till Race:_____

TODAY'S GOALS

Distance:

Speed:

Other:

THE RUN

Route:

Weather Conditions:

Time Start: Time End: Total Time:

Total Distance: Avg. Pace:

NOTES/THOUGHTS:

Date:_____ Days Till Race:_____

TODAY'S GOALS

Distance:

Speed:

Other:

THE RUN

Route:

Weather Conditions:

Time Start: Time End: Total Time:

Total Distance: Avg. Pace:

NOTES/THOUGHTS:

Date:_____ Days Till Race:_____

TODAY'S GOALS

Distance:

Speed:

Other:

THE RUN

Route:

Weather Conditions:

Time Start: Time End: Total Time:

Total Distance: Avg. Pace:

NOTES/THOUGHTS:

Date:_____ Days Till Race:_____

TODAY'S GOALS

Distance:

Speed:

Other:

THE RUN

Route:

Weather Conditions:

Time Start: Time End: Total Time:

Total Distance: Avg. Pace:

NOTES/THOUGHTS:

Date:_____ Days Till Race:_____

TODAY'S GOALS

Distance:

Speed:

Other:

THE RUN

Route:

Weather Conditions:

Time Start: Time End: Total Time:

Total Distance: Avg. Pace:

NOTES/THOUGHTS:

Date:_____ Days Till Race:_____

TODAY'S GOALS

Distance:

Speed:

Other:

THE RUN

Route:

Weather Conditions:

Time Start: Time End: Total Time:

Total Distance: Avg. Pace:

NOTES/THOUGHTS:

Date:_____ Days Till Race:_____

TODAY'S GOALS

Distance:

Speed:

Other:

THE RUN

Route:

Weather Conditions:

Time Start: Time End: Total Time:

Total Distance: Avg. Pace:

NOTES/THOUGHTS:

Date:_____ Days Till Race:_____

TODAY'S GOALS

Distance:

Speed:

Other:

THE RUN

Route:

Weather Conditions:

Time Start: Time End: Total Time:

Total Distance: Avg. Pace:

NOTES/THOUGHTS:

Date:_____ Days Till Race:_____

TODAY'S GOALS

Distance:

Speed:

Other:

THE RUN

Route:

Weather Conditions:

Time Start: Time End: Total Time:

Total Distance: Avg. Pace:

NOTES/THOUGHTS:

Date:_____ Days Till Race:_____

TODAY'S GOALS

Distance:

Speed:

Other:

THE RUN

Route:

Weather Conditions:

Time Start: Time End: Total Time:

Total Distance: Avg. Pace:

NOTES/THOUGHTS:

Date:_____ Days Till Race:_____

TODAY'S GOALS

Distance:

Speed:

Other:

THE RUN

Route:

Weather Conditions:

Time Start: Time End: Total Time:

Total Distance: Avg. Pace:

NOTES/THOUGHTS:

Date:_____ Days Till Race:_____

TODAY'S GOALS

Distance:

Speed:

Other:

THE RUN

Route:

Weather Conditions:

Time Start: Time End: Total Time:

Total Distance: Avg. Pace:

NOTES/THOUGHTS:

Date:_____ Days Till Race:_____

TODAY'S GOALS

Distance:

Speed:

Other:

THE RUN

Route:

Weather Conditions:

Time Start: Time End: Total Time:

Total Distance: Avg. Pace:

NOTES/THOUGHTS:

Date:_____ Days Till Race:_____

TODAY'S GOALS

Distance:

Speed:

Other:

THE RUN

Route:

Weather Conditions:

Time Start: Time End: Total Time:

Total Distance: Avg. Pace:

NOTES/THOUGHTS:

Date:_____ Days Till Race:_____

TODAY'S GOALS

Distance:

Speed:

Other:

THE RUN

Route:

Weather Conditions:

Time Start: Time End: Total Time:

Total Distance: Avg. Pace:

NOTES/THOUGHTS:

Date:_____ Days Till Race:_____

TODAY'S GOALS

Distance:

Speed:

Other:

THE RUN

Route:

Weather Conditions:

Time Start: Time End: Total Time:

Total Distance: Avg. Pace:

NOTES/THOUGHTS:

Date:_____ Days Till Race:_____

TODAY'S GOALS

Distance:

Speed:

Other:

THE RUN

Route:

Weather Conditions:

Time Start: Time End: Total Time:

Total Distance: Avg. Pace:

NOTES/THOUGHTS:

Date:_____ Days Till Race:_____

TODAY'S GOALS

Distance:

Speed:

Other:

THE RUN

Route:

Weather Conditions:

Time Start: Time End: Total Time:

Total Distance: Avg. Pace:

NOTES/THOUGHTS:

Date:_____ Days Till Race:_____

TODAY'S GOALS

Distance:

Speed:

Other:

THE RUN

Route:

Weather Conditions:

Time Start: Time End: Total Time:

Total Distance: Avg. Pace:

NOTES/THOUGHTS:

Date:_____ Days Till Race:_____

TODAY'S GOALS

Distance:

Speed:

Other:

THE RUN

Route:

Weather Conditions:

Time Start: Time End: Total Time:

Total Distance: Avg. Pace:

NOTES/THOUGHTS:

Date:_____ Days Till Race:_____

TODAY'S GOALS

Distance:

Speed:

Other:

THE RUN

Route:

Weather Conditions:

Time Start: Time End: Total Time:

Total Distance: Avg. Pace:

NOTES/THOUGHTS:

Date:_____ Days Till Race:_____

TODAY'S GOALS

Distance:

Speed:

Other:

THE RUN

Route:

Weather Conditions:

Time Start: Time End: Total Time:

Total Distance: Avg. Pace:

NOTES/THOUGHTS:

Date:_____ Days Till Race:_____

TODAY'S GOALS

Distance:

Speed:

Other:

THE RUN

Route:

Weather Conditions:

Time Start: Time End: Total Time:

Total Distance: Avg. Pace:

NOTES/THOUGHTS:

Date:_____ Days Till Race:_____

TODAY'S GOALS

Distance:

Speed:

Other:

THE RUN

Route:

Weather Conditions:

Time Start: Time End: Total Time:

Total Distance: Avg. Pace:

NOTES/THOUGHTS:

Date:_____ Days Till Race:_____

TODAY'S GOALS

Distance:

Speed:

Other:

THE RUN

Route:

Weather Conditions:

Time Start: Time End: Total Time:

Total Distance: Avg. Pace:

NOTES/THOUGHTS:

Date:_____ Days Till Race:_____

TODAY'S GOALS

Distance:

Speed:

Other:

THE RUN

Route:

Weather Conditions:

Time Start: Time End: Total Time:

Total Distance: Avg. Pace:

NOTES/THOUGHTS:

Date:_____ Days Till Race:_____

TODAY'S GOALS

Distance:

Speed:

Other:

THE RUN

Route:

Weather Conditions:

Time Start: Time End: Total Time:

Total Distance: Avg. Pace:

NOTES/THOUGHTS:

Date:_____ Days Till Race:_____

TODAY'S GOALS

Distance:

Speed:

Other:

THE RUN

Route:

Weather Conditions:

Time Start: Time End: Total Time:

Total Distance: Avg. Pace:

NOTES/THOUGHTS:

Date:_____ Days Till Race:_____

TODAY'S GOALS

Distance:

Speed:

Other:

THE RUN

Route:

Weather Conditions:

Time Start: Time End: Total Time:

Total Distance: Avg. Pace:

NOTES/THOUGHTS:

Date:_____ Days Till Race:_____

TODAY'S GOALS

Distance:

Speed:

Other:

THE RUN

Route:

Weather Conditions:

Time Start: Time End: Total Time:

Total Distance: Avg. Pace:

NOTES/THOUGHTS:

Date:_____ Days Till Race:_____

TODAY'S GOALS

Distance:

Speed:

Other:

THE RUN

Route:

Weather Conditions:

Time Start: Time End: Total Time:

Total Distance: Avg. Pace:

NOTES/THOUGHTS:

Date:_____ Days Till Race:_____

TODAY'S GOALS

Distance:

Speed:

Other:

THE RUN

Route:

Weather Conditions:

Time Start: Time End: Total Time:

Total Distance: Avg. Pace:

NOTES/THOUGHTS:

REFLECTION

REFLECTION

REFLECTION

REFLECTION

www.ingramcontent.com/pod-product-compliance
Lightning Source LLC
Chambersburg PA
CBHW051038030426
42336CB00015B/2937